50 Consecutive Pushups
--
Ultimate Calisthenics Challenge

Jacob Eckhardt

Copyright © 2014 by Jacob B. Eckhardt

All rights reserved. This book or any portion thereof
may not be reproduced or used in any manner whatsoever
without the express written permission of the publisher
except for the use of brief quotations in a book review.
Printed in the United States of America

First Printing, 2014

ISBN: 978-1502857989

www.CalisthenicsTribe.com

Photos by: Andrea Eckhardt

Cover Art: Somiron Mandal

Table of Contents

Preface 1

Chapter 0 - Ground Zero 9

Chapter 1 - Level 1 19

Chapter 2 - Level 2 26

Chapter 3 - Level 3 35

Chapter 4 - Level 4 45

Chapter 5 - Level 5 53

Preface

You've probably witnessed people engaging in push-up contests to try and outdo their friends. The winner always gets a cheer from the crowd, seemingly becoming a hero in the minute-long contest. Being able to perform many push-ups is simply one of the greatest feats of strength.

Why do you want to do push-ups? I mean they are used as military punishment for goodness sake, and you want to do them voluntarily? What is wrong with you?!

I'm only kidding of course because back when I first started trying to get in shape, I couldn't do a single push-up. My arms would shake as if the floor was an evil massage pad, and I'd lower myself to an immediate collapse. Whether you're at that stage or a little farther ahead, there's something in this book to help everyone improve in both push-ups and general fitness.

The push-up is the ultimate test of what kind of physical condition you are in. If anyone were silly enough to question your strength, the push-up test would be the easiest and quickest way to show them you're the boss. It tests the whole body, activating muscle groups in the chest, shoulders, arms, back, abs, hips, and legs.

If you are interested in calisthenics, this program is exactly what you need to give you a good calisthenics base since push-ups build strength in the entire body. If you aren't able to do 50 push-ups, you are going to struggle doing any kind of calisthenic exercise. You really need that good base of strength first.

Since you're reading this right now, I'm going to assume you can't do very many push-ups, which is totally fine! Most people can't, but you're ahead of most people because you're here trying to fix that. In mere weeks, I'm going to bring you from your current push-up ability and take you to a whole new level–50 consecutive push-ups.

You might be wondering how the hell you're going to do that, and that's why I'm here. I'm going to ensure you make it all the way there by giving you the best workouts, video explanations, and full support along the way. I'm a certified personal trainer by the National Academy of Sports Medicine and have worked with right around 100 clients in a commercial gym. Most of my clients wanted to do a lot of bodyweight exercises that they could then practice at home as well, so of course, I had them doing push-ups. They all made significant progress, and you could see significant differences in their bodies after 4-8 weeks, especially in the arms.

I saw a need for this kind of program because all of the push-up routines out there simply tell you to just do more push-ups every week. Really? Not only could anyone think that up on their own, but it also won't get anybody very far. That's why I've included many progressive variations of push-ups and other exercises that help strengthen the main muscles used, giving you maximum results in the shortest amount of time.

The best part? It will only take you 20 minutes, 3 times a week. That's less than 1% of your total time spent awake over the course of a week! Since the workouts are short, you should be giving a maximum effort each time, really concentrating on each rep and grinding out the tough ones. Some of you may be tempted to do the workouts more than 3 times a week, but doing that is going to hold you back. Your muscles are built while you are resting and recovering, so doing push-ups every day would interrupt that process. Your only goal should be to give it a maximum effort those 3 days a week, and rest during the designated rest days.

If you have a question about anything at all, just visit my website at www.CalisthenicsTribe.com and click "Ask Jake," and I will answer it as soon as I can.

Also, along the way, you guys will earn badges for every level you complete. Motivation is one of the toughest parts when it comes to keeping a consistent workout schedule, so I want you guys to have something to work towards. If you register on the website, you can request the badges for completing each level, and the community will be able to see them in your profile. There is also an activity feed that immediately shows everyone you earned the badge, so show everyone what you've got and try to compete with the other members!

While getting to 50 push-ups is the main goal here, that's not all this program is about. When you've finished this book, you will feel amazing–you'll literally be a brand new person. Because aside from improving your strength and fitness level, this program has other amazing benefits as well.

- You will feel more energized.
- You will have a more attractive body.
- You will have much better posture.
- You will have more self-confidence.
- You will have more self-discipline.
- You will have learned how to eat healthier.

Posture Improvements

One thing I want to talk a bit about in particular is posture improvements. If you have a hunched back or your head protrudes forward, the push-up will train your muscles to correct that and start to bring everything back in line. Push-ups are going to help strengthen the muscles that support you and give you a nice stout frame.

In order to see these posture improvements, focus on keeping your neck held back during the exercises. Try to make a "double-chin," by retracting your neck backwards. You should be able to feel some muscles working to keep your head there when doing so, and keeping that position during exercise will strengthen those muscles that are supposed to keep your head in line with your spine. Video #1 in the video library on my website www.CalisthenicsTribe.com teaches this in more detail.

Anyone Can Make Amazing Progress

I, personally, was the really skinny guy with no muscle, and I was just generally weak. However, it doesn't matter whether you are man, woman, skinny, average-sized, or overweight–all of you will make progress.

One thing I would like to state is that if you are overweight or have some extra pounds, you will progress much quicker if you start on a healthy weight loss diet. Every extra pound of fat you have is like a brick tied to your body that's going to make it that much harder to do a push-up or any exercise for that matter.

The good news is, people who are overweight are generally stronger than the skinnier ones, so losing fat while gaining strength will bring quick progress in this program.

I wrote up a free sample diet plan for both men and women to help get you guys started if you want to burn off some of that stubborn fat. It's kind of long and I didn't want to take up too much room in this book with it, so if you're interested, just visit the website and click on "Diet Plans" at the top. It tells you how many calories you should eat, and I list out how many grams of fat, carbs, and protein are in each food and the total counts.

I really, really want you all to succeed in achieving your goals because fitness has made such a huge impact on my life, and I want other people to experience the benefits as well. So please, if you have any questions or concerns, I want you to contact me.

Attacking the Muscle from Both Angles

In this program, we are attacking your muscles from 2 angles: (1) We are adding strength to them (Monday and Friday workouts). (2) We are increasing muscular endurance so you can use that strength to its maximum potential and perform more reps before your muscles get tired (Wednesday workouts). Think of it as cardio for your muscles.

As a result, your muscles are going to become bigger and more defined as well. Training both ways is going to give you maximum progress in the shortest amount of time.

Universal Form for Push-Ups

The form will be slightly different for each exercise, which I will explain in the text, pictures and video when the times comes to do them, but there are two rules that apply to all types of push-ups.

Rule #1: Your butt, back, and neck have to form a straight line. Keep your back tight and straight, and especially avoid letting it arch. If you are going for that last push-up and your form breaks down causing your back to arch, you should stop immediately. Trying to force it could result in a back injury. Likewise, don't lift your butt up into the air and bring it out of line because this will make the push-up easier, and it won't count as a real one.

Rule #2: Full Range of Motion – Lowering yourself all the way down for the push-up means your nose is about an inch from the ground at the bottom. Don't cheat yourself by only going down halfway because that's not going to activate every muscle involved, and as a result, you won't progress very quickly in strength.

Note that some exercises will require slightly different hand placement and lowering techniques, which will be explained as they come.

Please read through each level in its entirety before performing the workouts. It will greatly help in understanding exactly what you need to do.

*Tip: If you get lost or confused on the formatting, you can look at the template at the end of each level. It's a sample plan for someone who would be running through these workouts. It shows you exactly what someone may be doing, although you may be able to level up faster than the template I laid out. I anticipate most of you will!

Getting Started

First of all, I know not all of you are at the same level, so some of you may be starting at the very beginning while some might be stuck at X number of push-ups. This book progresses you through levels based on how many push-ups you can do, so first figure out what level you are going to be starting in.

Ground Zero – You are in Ground Zero if you can't do 1 single push-up.
Level 1 – If you can do 1 push-up but can't do 10, you are at Level 1.
Level 2 – If you can do 10 push-ups but can't do 20, you are at Level 2.
Level 3 – If you can do 20 push-ups but can't do 30, you are at Level 3.
Level 4 – If you can do 30 push-ups but can't do 40, you are at Level 4.
Level 5 – If you can do 40 push-ups but can't do 50, you are at Level 5.

Level 5 is where you hit the 50 push-up mark. When you qualify to start at a higher level, you can still collect the badges from the previous levels. For example, if you can do 25 push-ups consecutively, you are in Level 3. Therefore, you can collect your Ground Zero and Level 1 & 2 badges. Simply head over to www.CalisthenicsTribe.com to collect them.

Throughout the book, you will be utilizing a maximum effort set. I call it a **"BOOM"** set, and you're going to be using these record-busting sets almost every workout. Basically, all it means is that you are going to failure whenever you see a BOOM set in your workout. You will want to set a new record for your BOOM set every time you do the workouts; this is how you progress.

Now, let's get started!

Chapter 0 - Ground Zero

Alright, we're at Ground Zero for those of you who are really having a hard time with any type of push-up. Don't worry though, you'll be out of ground zero in no time.

The first thing you need to do is find somewhere to do incline push-ups. Having your body on an incline is going to make it easier, and we will use a smaller and smaller angle to get you to a flat push-up.

Method

Step 1 – Find a wall or counter where you can perform incline push-ups. Here is the form:

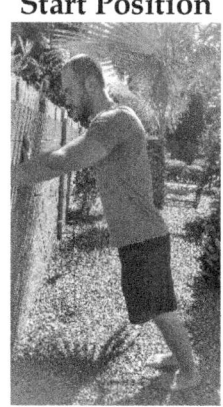

Start Position

(Hands just outside shoulder width at chest level)

End Position

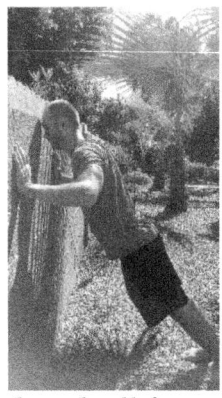

(Butt, back, and neck all form a straight line)

Step 2 – Ok, so you've seen the form, now you just need to find the right places to do the rep ranges. In the workouts coming up, you will be doing sets of 5, sets of 10, and sets of 15 incline push-ups. So you will be using three different angles, and the first one you need to figure out is the 15 rep starting point.

As you can see from the pictures above, I am against a wall with a high angle. Maybe you will need a higher angle, but first you just need to find an angle where you can perform **18** incline push-ups. Those 18 should be pretty difficult and should only leave you with 1-2 more left in the tank. Why 18? You will be doing 5 sets of 15 push-ups, so finding the 18 rep mark will ensure you are able to do 15 reps 5 times.

Step 3 – You got your 15 rep starting point in the last step. Now you need to do this with your 10 rep starting point. Find an angle that only allows you to do **12-13** reps with 1-2 left in the tank. This angle will be lower than in step 2. For example, maybe now you use a kitchen counter instead of a wall.

Step 4 – Lastly, find the angle where you can only do **6-7** reps with 1 left in the tank. This will be the lowest angle, and it marks your 5 rep starting point. A possible home object for this angle would be something like a coffee table.

Take note of these 3 starting points, because you will be using them in the coming workouts.

*Tip: If this has you confused, check out video #2 in the video library on www.CalisthenicsTribe.com. It's much easier to explain and show over video than it is just text.

Ok, great, you've figured out your 5, 10, and 15 rep starting points. Now, you're going to have a workout 3 times a week. Here's what a full 7-days should look like.

Monday - Incline Push-ups 3x5 and Incline Push-ups 5x10
Tuesday - Off
Wednesday - 3x8 Negatives and Incline Push-ups 5x15
Thursday - Off
Friday – Incline Push-ups 3x5 and Incline Push-ups 5x10
Saturday - Off
Sunday - Off

Now, if you are totally new to working out, you might not understand what I just wrote, so let me break it down. "Incline Push-ups 3x5" means you will perform 3 sets of incline push-ups for 5 reps. A set consists of repetitions. So 3 sets of 5 reps looks like this:

Set 1: 5 reps
Set 2: 5 reps
Set 3: 5 reps

And then move on to the next exercise.

The Monday and Friday workouts are always the same in each level, except for the difficulty. (Keep in mind you can pick your own days of the week, but please keep the same structure)

Incline Push-ups 3x5's and 5x10's Workout (Monday and Friday)

Alright, you've got your 5 rep starting point; here's how this workout is going to go. You're going to do the first 2 sets of 5, and then on the last set, you should be getting as many as you can, and I emphasize only on the last set. These are the "BOOM" sets that I was talking about.

You do the same thing for the 5x10's as well. Get your 4 sets of 10, and then BOOM out as many as you can on the last set. Remember to keep good form — don't force out a push-up with bad form just to be able to say you did a higher number. Bad push-ups don't count.

BOOMing as many as you can on that last set is what's going to give you maximum progression. It's a term called progressive overload, which is vital for muscle and strength gain. It means you should be trying to do better on each workout than you did on the last one.

When you perform the same workout again a few days later, you have to try and outdo however many you did during your last workout of 3x5's and 5x10's. You want to try and demolish your last record by getting as many as you can on that last BOOM set.

This means you have to write it down every time, otherwise you're bound to forget. If you got 6 on the last set of 5's in the first workout, you should be aiming to squash that record and get at least 7 on your next attempt. Tell yourself you're gonna do it, and grind out those last reps. Those last reps are the ones that cause you to improve, so give it all you've got!

This workout is what improves your strength the most. Those first 3 sets of 5 reps are strength builders, and the 5x10's have hybrid benefits, meaning they increase strength a little bit and increase muscular endurance a little bit, too. This workout generally shouldn't take more than about 20 minutes.

Now, once you are able to do 8 reps on the final set of the 3x5's, you are ready to increase the difficulty. Lower the angle of the push-up until you find that it's hard to hit 5 reps again. I explain this concept clearly in video #3.

Negatives and 5x15's Workout (Wednesday)

Negatives are when you lower yourself down for the push-up really slowly. When you aren't yet able push yourself back up, this is how we are going to help build strength and stabilization. So all you have to do is lower yourself to the floor as slowly as you can until you collapse. Once you collapse, just reset and go back to the starting position. If you aren't able to position yourself in the full push-up position to start the negative, it's no problem—just do negatives from an incline position.

For this workout, you are just going to do 3 sets of 8 negatives. You are not trying to increase on the last set for negatives—no boom sets here. Just get all 3 sets of 8 and you're good to go. Next, use your 15 rep starting point that I had you write down from earlier. And again, you are going to get as many as you can on the last set. Performing 15 reps is going to increase your muscular endurance.

Every time you do the 5x15's workout, you should increase the difficulty (lower the angle) just a little bit. If you increase the difficulty a little too much and find you can't get 15 reps on all 5 sets, that's totally fine! Just write down however many you were able to do and try to beat that next time.

Final Sets

I know I said this already, but I really want to stress how important it is that you give it your all on those final sets. You've gotta go for the freakin' gold here. Hype yourself up and tell yourself you're going to destroy your record from last time, and then prove it to yourself. Blow your previous record out of the water like a BOSS.

Rest Periods

Monday and Friday Workout
1.5-2 minutes between sets for the 3x5 incline push-ups
1-1.5 minutes between sets for the 5x10 incline push-ups

Wednesday Workout
1.5 minutes between sets for the negatives
1-1.5 minutes between sets for the 5x15 incline push-ups

Ground Zero Completion Requirement: 1 full push-up

Ground Zero Sample Plan

Week 1

Day			
1	Incline Push-ups Set 1: 5 Set 2: 5 BOOM: 5		Incline Push-ups Set 1: 10 Set 2: 10 Set 3: 10 Set 4: 10 BOOM: 10
2	Negatives Set 1: 8 Set 2: 8 Set 3: 8		Incline Push-ups Set 1: 15 Set 2: 15 Set 3: 15 Set 4: 15 Set 5: 15
3	Incline Push-ups Set 1: 5 Set 2: 5 BOOM: 6 *New Record*		Incline Push-ups Set 1: 10 Set 2: 10 Set 3: 10 Set 4: 10 BOOM: 11 *New Record*

Week 2

Day		
1	Incline Push-ups Set 1: 5 Set 2: 5 BOOM: 7 *New Record*	Incline Push-ups Set 1: 10 Set 2: 10 Set 3: 10 Set 4: 10 BOOM: 12 *New Record*
2	Negatives Set 1: 8 Set 2: 8 Set 3: 8	Increased Difficulty Incline Push-ups Set 1: 15 Set 2: 15 Set 3: 15 Set 4: 15 Set 5: 15
3	Incline Push-ups Set 1: 5 Set 2: 5 BOOM: 8 *New Record*	Incline Push-ups Set 1: 10 Set 2: 10 Set 3: 10 Set 4: 10 BOOM: 13 *New Record*

Week 3

Day			
1	Increased Difficulty Incline Push-ups Set 1: 5 Set 2: 5 BOOM: 5		Incline Push-ups Set 1: 10 Set 2: 10 Set 3: 10 Set 4: 10 BOOM: 14 *New Record*
2	Negatives Set 1: 8 Set 2: 8 Set 3: 8		Increased Difficulty Incline Push-ups Set 1: 15 Set 2: 15 Set 3: 15 Set 4: 15 Set 5: 15
3	Incline Push-ups Set 1: 5 Set 2: 5 BOOM: 6 *New Record*		Incline Push-ups Set 1: 10 Set 2: 10 Set 3: 10 Set 4: 10 BOOM: 15 *New Record*

Week 4

Day			
1	Incline Push-ups Set 1: 5 Set 2: 5 BOOM: 8 *New Record*		Incline Push-ups Set 1: 10 Set 2: 10 Set 3: 10 Set 4: 10 BOOM: 17 *New Record*
2	Negatives Set 1: 8 Set 2: 8 BOOM: 8		Increased Difficulty Incline Push-ups Set 1: 15 Set 2: 15 Set 3: 15 Set 4: 15 Set 5: 15
3	Increased Difficulty Incline Push-ups Set 1: 5 Set 2: 5 BOOM: 5		Incline Push-ups Set 1: 10 Set 2: 10 Set 3: 10 Set 4: 10 BOOM: 18 *New Record*

Chapter 1 - Level 1

If you're here, you've passed Ground Zero! Head over to www.CalisthenicsTribe.com and claim your Ground Zero badge! You just have to sign up, and on your profile just click that you completed Ground Zero, and I will approve you for the badge! Here's to many more to come!

Since you're a seasoned veteran, we will just jump right into the workouts.

Level 1 Workouts
Monday - Max push-ups+incline push-ups (3 sets of 10 total reps) + 3x8 Negatives
Tuesday - Off
Wednesday - 5x15's and 3 Static Holds
Thursday - Off
Friday - Max push-ups+incline push-ups (3 sets of 10 total reps) + 3x8 Negatives
Saturday - Off
Sunday - Off

Max/Incline Push-Ups+Negatives Workout (Monday and Friday)

For the first set of push-ups, you are going to do as many full push-ups as you can, and then once you can't do any more, immediately drop down to knee push-ups and make your way up to 10 total reps.

For example, if you did 1 full push-up, and couldn't do another, you would immediately do 9 small-angled incline push-ups (i.e. using a coffee table) for a total of 10. You will do this for 3 sets. On your second set you may not even be able to get 1 full push-up, but that's 100% fine and expected in many cases, so in that case just do 10 incline push-ups.

You should again be trying to improve every time you do this workout, trying to add more full push-ups every time. Check out video #4 over on calisthenicstribe.com to see exactly what I mean.

Regular Push-up

Start Position

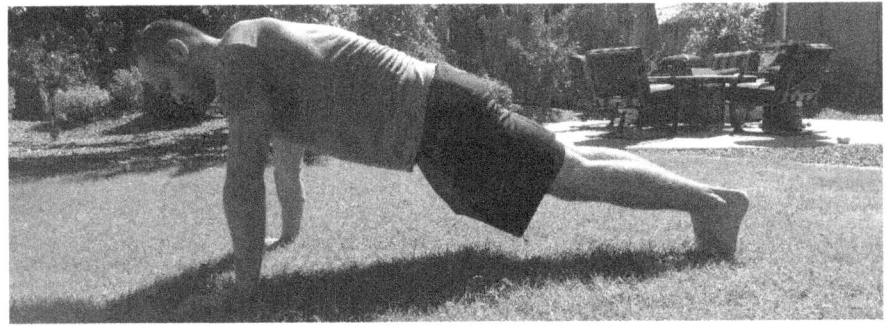

(Hands are just outside shoulder width)

End Position

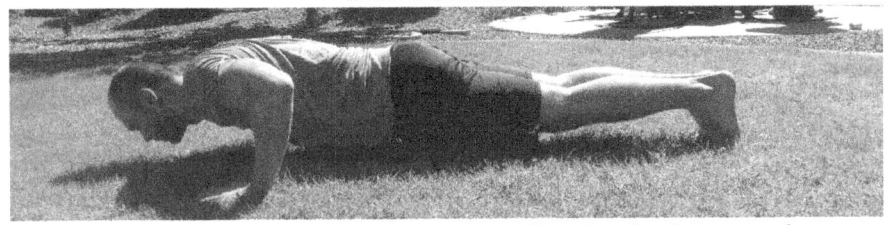

(Back stays straight. Keep neck in line by looking at the ground, not up)

Now for the negatives, you just do the same thing as in Ground Zero (If you have skipped to this point, please refer to Chapter 1 on how to do negatives). Lower yourself as slowly as possible for 8 reps. If it's getting pretty easy for you to do this, you can wear a backpack and put something inside to weigh you down. When I do them, I just use textbooks or fresh stacks of printer paper. Make sure the straps are snug, otherwise the backpack will slip a little bit. Again, you are performing 3 sets.

3 Static Holds and 5x15's (Wednesday)

Static holds are somewhat similar to a negative, except once you get halfway down, you hold it there for as long as you can. Make sure you time yourself and write it down every time because next time you do the workout you will want to beat your total time. You'll do the static hold 3 times, so you would add up the 3 times and try to beat that next week. Watch video #5 on the website for clarification.

We are still using the 5x15's to build up some muscular endurance, so find an incline push-up position that allows you to achieve those 5 sets of 15 reps.

Rest Periods

Monday and Friday Workout
1.5-2 minutes for the Full/Incline push-up combo
1-1.5 minutes for the negatives

Wednesday Workout
1-1.5 minutes for the 5x15's
1.5 minutes for the static holds

Level 1 Completion Requirement: 10 full push-ups

Level 1 Sample Plan

Week 1

Day	Exercise 1		Exercise 2
1	**Full/Incline Push-ups** Set 1: 1 Full + 9 Incline Set 2: 1 Full + 9 Incline Set 3: 0 Full + 10 Incline		**Weighted Negatives** Set 1: 8 Set 2: 8 Set 3: 8
2	**Increased Difficulty** Incline Push-ups Set 1: 15 Set 2: 15 Set 3: 15 Set 4: 15 Set 5: 15		Static Holds Set 1: 10s Set 2: 8s Set 3: 7s Total: 25s
3	*New Record* Full/Incline Push-ups Set 1: 2 Full + 8 Incline Set 2: 2 Full + 8 Incline Set 3: 1 Full + 9 Incline		**Weighted Negatives** Set 1: 8 Set 2: 8 Set 3: 8

Week 2

Day	Exercise 1		Exercise 2
1	*New Record* Full/Incline Push-ups Set 1: 3 Full + 7 Incline Set 2: 2 Full + 8 Incline Set 3: 2 Full + 8 Incline		**Weighted Negatives** Set 1: 8 Set 2: 8 Set 3: 8
2	Increased Difficulty Incline Push-ups Set 1: 15 Set 2: 15 Set 3: 15 Set 4: 15 Set 5: 15		Static Holds Set 1: 15s Set 2: 12s Set 3: 10s Total: 37s *New Record*
3	*New Record* Full/Incline Push-ups Set 1: 5 Full + 5 Incline Set 2: 4 Full + 6 Incline Set 3: 3 Full + 7 Incline		**Weighted Negatives** Set 1: 8 Set 2: 8 Set 3: 8

Week 3

Day	Exercise 1		Exercise 2
1	*New Record* Full/Incline Push-ups Set 1: 6 Full + 4 Incline Set 2: 5 Full + 5 Incline Set 3: 4 Full + 6 Incline		**Weighted Negatives** Set 1: 8 Set 2: 8 Set 3: 8
2	Increased Difficulty Incline Push-ups Set 1: 15 Set 2: 15 Set 3: 15 Set 4: 15 Set 5: 15		Static Holds Set 1: 20s Set 2: 15s Set 3: 13s Total: 48s *New Record*
3	*New Record* Full/Incline Push-ups Set 1: 7 Full + 3 Incline Set 2: 6 Full + 4 Incline Set 3: 5 Full + 5 Incline		**Weighted Negatives** Set 1: 8 Set 2: 8 Set 3: 8

Week 4

Day	Exercise 1		Exercise 2
1	*New Record* Full/Incline Push-ups Set 1: 8 Full + 2 Incline Set 2: 7 Full + 3 Incline Set 3: 6 Full + 4 Incline		**Weighted Negatives** Set 2: 8 Set 3: 8
2	Increased Difficulty Incline Push-ups Set 1: 15 Set 2: 15 Set 3: 15 Set 4: 15 Set 5: 15		Static Holds Set 1: 27s Set 2: 22s Set 3: 17s Total: 66s *New Record*
3	*New Record* Full/Incline Push-ups Set 1: **10 FULL PUSH-UPS!** Set 2: 8 Full + 2 Incline Set 3: 7 Full + 3 Incline *Pass*		**Weighted Negatives** Set 1: 8 Set 2: 8 Set 3: 8

Chapter 2 - Level 2

Badge Don't forget to head over to the website and grab your level 1 badge!

Level 2 Workouts

Monday - 8/8/BOOM + Tricep Dips 6/6/BOOM
Tuesday - Off
Wednesday - Incline Push-ups 5x20 and 3 Weighted Static Holds
Thursday - Off
Friday - 8/8/BOOM + Tricep Dips 6/6/BOOM
Saturday - Off
Sunday - Off

Push-ups 8/8/BOOM + Tricep Dips 6/6/BOOM (Monday and Friday)

Alright, we're kicking it up a notch here. After passing Level 1 with 10 push-ups, you should be able to do 2 sets of 8 reps and then a BOOM set in which you attempt to get as many as you can.

Now, this week we are adding in some tricep dips that are going to help you with some arm strength. Triceps are one of the main muscles used in push-ups, so we want to strengthen them up and improve your all-around strength as much as possible. With these, try to stop 1 rep short of failure. Your failure point will increase every week as you get stronger, so you should still be doing more reps every week, just like in the sample plan. To do these, you will only need a chair.

Tricep Dips
Start Position

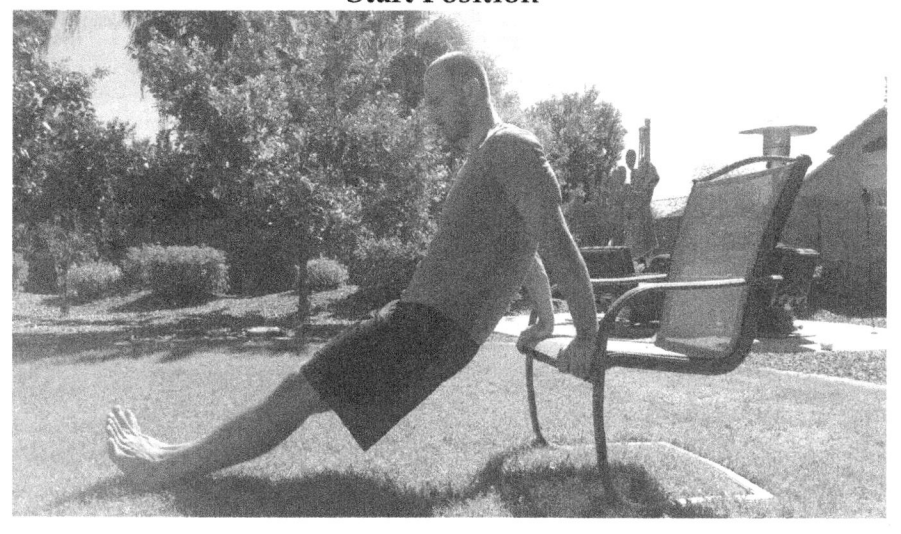

End Position

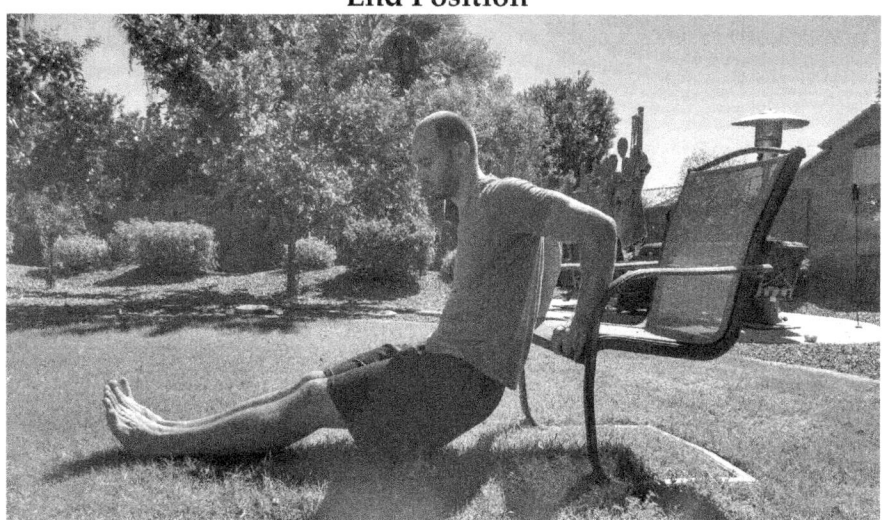

Bad End Position

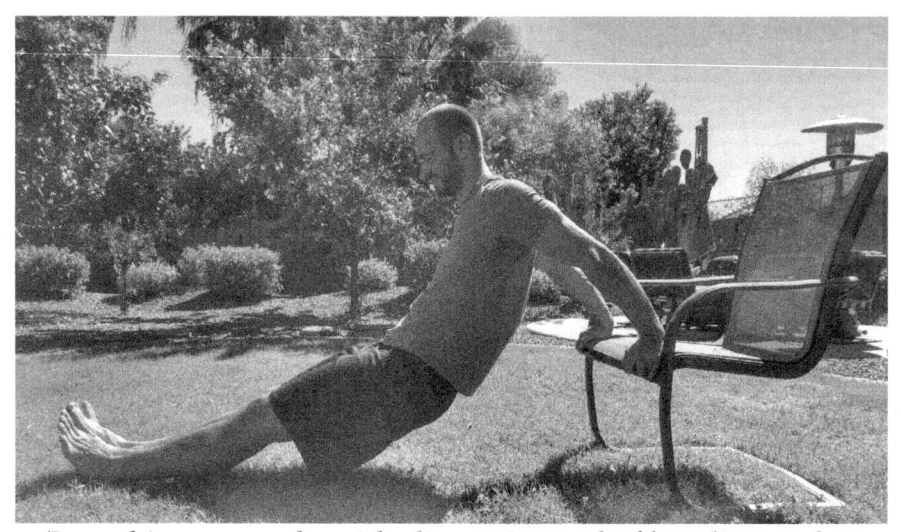

(I see this commonly with clients; Instead of bending at the elbows they fall forward with the shoulders. Avoid this!)

Check out the video #6 in the video library on www.CalisthenicsTribe.com where I clearly demonstrate the difference.

Incline Push-ups 5x20's and 3 Weighted Static Holds (Wednesday)

In Level 1 you were doing 5x15's and static holds, and this week you are just going to make them a bit harder. You will need to find a good incline level where you are able to push out 20 incline push-ups, which should be pretty similar to the incline you used for the 5x15's. The reason we are stepping it up to 20 is to increase muscular endurance.

Now, with the static holds, you will need to bust out a backpack. When you do the static holds, wear a backpack with some weight in it, something like 10-20 pounds. It doesn't have to be actual weights — like I said earlier I just use either textbooks or fresh stacks of printer paper. Perform the static holds just as you did in the last level. (For this who have started in this level, refer to video #5 for instruction on how to do static holds.)

Weighted Static Holds
Start Position

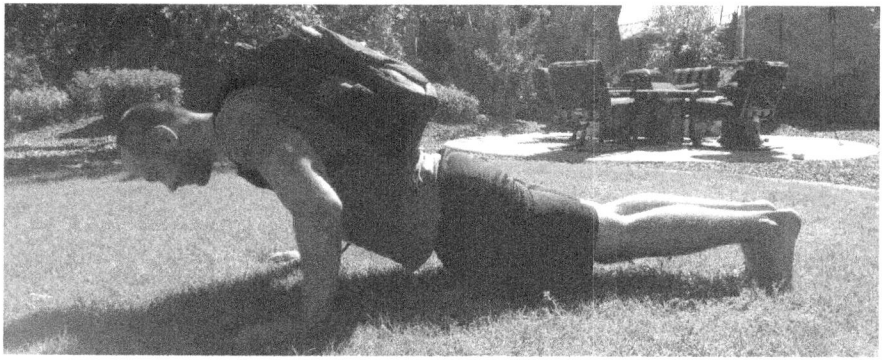

(Just like the other static holds. Arms bent about half way and hold)

End Position
(Again no proper end position. Just hold until you collapse)

Rest Periods

Monday and Friday Workout
1.5-2 minutes for the 3x8 push-ups
1.5 minutes for the tricep dips

Wednesday Workout
1.5 minutes for the 5x20 incline push-ups
1.5 minutes for the weighted static holds

Level 2 Completion Requirement: 20 full push-ups

Level 2 Sample Plan

Week 1

Day	Exercise 1	Exercise 2
1	Push-ups Set 1: 8 Set 2: 8 BOOM: 8	Tricep Dips Set 1: 6 Set 2: 6 Set 3: 6
2	Incline Push-ups Set 1: 20 Set 2: 20 Set 3: 20 Set 4: 20 Set 5: 20	Weighted Static Holds Set 1: 15s Set 2: 10s Set 3: 9s Total: **34s**
3	Push-ups Set 1: 8 Set 2: 8 BOOM: 10 *New Record*	Tricep Dips Set 1: 6 Set 2: 6 Set 3: 8 *New Record*

Week 2

Day	Exercise 1	Exercise 2
1	Push-ups Set 1: 8 Set 2: 8 BOOM: 12 *New Record*	Tricep Dips Set 1: 6 Set 2: 6 Set 3: 10 *New Record*
2	Increased Difficulty Incline Push-ups Set 1: 20 Set 2: 20 Set 3: 20 Set 4: 20 Set 5: 20	Weighted Static Holds Set 1: 20s Set 2: 15s Set 3: 13s Total: **51s** *New Record*
3	Push-ups Set 1: 8 Set 2: 8 BOOM: 14 *New Record*	Tricep Dips Set 1: 6 Set 2: 6 Set 3: 11 *New Record*

Week 3

Day	Exercise 1		Exercise 2
1	Push-ups Set 1: 8 Set 2: 8 BOOM: 15 *New Record*		Added Weight Tricep Dips Set 1: 6 Set 2: 6 Set 3: 6
2	Increased Difficulty Incline Push-ups Set 1: 20 Set 2: 20 Set 3: 20 Set 4: 20 Set 5: 20		Weighted Static Holds Set 1: 26s Set 2: 21s Set 3: 17s Total: **64s** *New Record*
3	Push-ups Set 1: 8 Set 2: 8 BOOM: 17 *New Record*		Tricep Dips Set 1: 6 Set 2: 6 Set 3: 8 *New Record*

Week 4

Day	Exercise 1		Exercise 2
1	Push-ups Set 1: 8 Set 2: 8 BOOM: 18 *New Record*		Tricep Dips Set 1: 6 Set 2: 6 Set 3: 10 *New Record*
2	Increased Difficulty Incline Push-ups Set 1: 20 Set 2: 20 Set 3: 20 Set 4: 20 Set 5: 20		Weighted Static Holds Set 1: 33s Set 2: 26s Set 3: 21s Total: **80s** *New Record*
3	Push-ups Set 1: 8 Set 2: 8 **BOOM: 20 FULL PUSH-UPS** *Pass*		Added Weight Tricep Dips Set 1: 6 Set 2: 6 Set 3: 6

Chapter 3 - Level 3

Badge Don't forget to hit the website and request your level 2 badge!

Level 3 Workouts

Monday - 6/6/BOOM Weighted Push-ups + Diamond Push-ups 8/8/BOOM
Tuesday - Off
Wednesday - BOOM/12/12/12/12 + Tricep Dips 8/8/BOOM
Thursday - Off
Friday - Weighted Push-ups 6/6/BOOM + Diamond Push-ups 8/8/BOOM
Saturday - Off
Sunday - Off

Alright, we're bringing out the big guns now. Weighted push-ups! You're going to break out the weighted backpack and whatever kind of weights you've been using once again.

Workout: Weighted Push-ups 6/6/BOOM + Diamond Push-ups 8/8/BOOM (Monday and Friday)

Alright, if you're at this point you're doing great! 20 push-ups is a great accomplishment, and now we've got to switch it up a little bit in order to push past 20. Since you can do so many push-ups now, the high reps aren't going to give you much strength anymore; we would be improving muscular endurance only, which as we said earlier will plateau our results eventually without strength training. Therefore, we need to add some weight, so hopefully you've got your backpack and makeshift weights ready to go!

<u>Weighted Push-ups</u>

These are the same as regular push-ups, except you will have a backpack on.

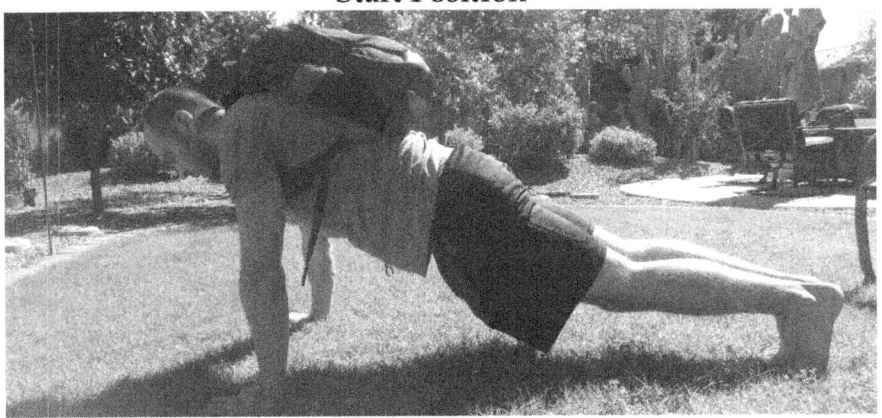

Start Position

End Position

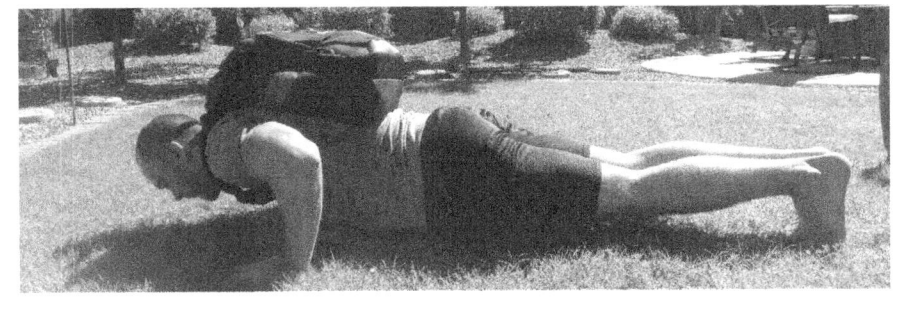

You will want to put enough weight in the backpack so that it's tough for you to get 6-8 reps with it. You are going to do these the same as all the other push-ups you've been doing, 6/6/BOOM style. Get your 2 sets of 6 at whatever weight is challenging enough for you, and then BOOM it out on the last set, grinding out as many as you can. Write it down, and improve on the next workout, rinse and repeat, you know the drill.

Also, once you hit 8 reps on the boom set, you should add more weight instead of going past 8 reps. With this workout, we are trying to add more strength which is better accomplished with more weight instead of reps.

<u>Diamond Push-ups</u>

We've got a new kind of push-up this week, the diamond push-up. Watch video #7 for the proper form.

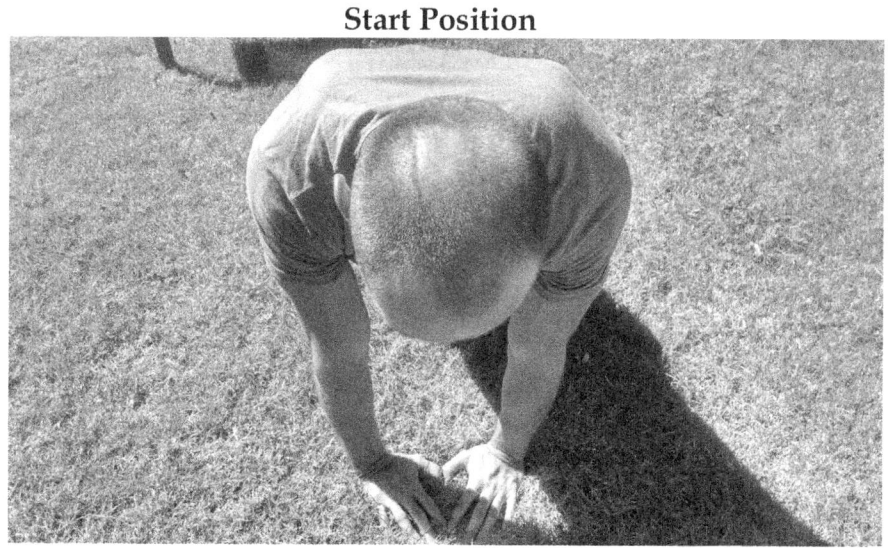

Start Position

(Only difference between these and regular push-ups is hand placement. Hands should form a diamond or heart)

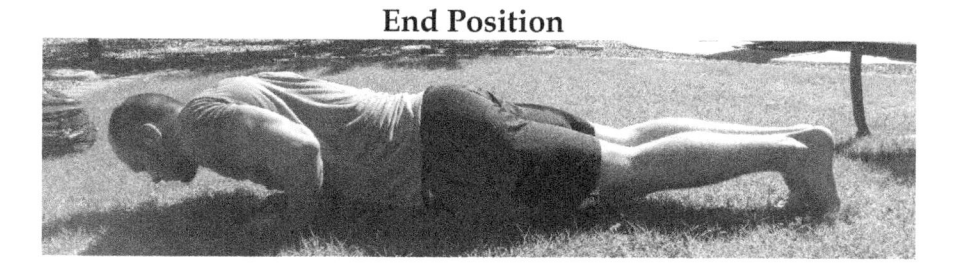

End Position

(Keep your elbows tucked in towards your torso as much as possible. Don't let the elbows flare out.)

Alright you've got the form down, now all you have to do is 3 sets of them. How many reps? That's going to vary. You will be tired from those first sets of weighted backpack push-ups so there's no way to definitively tell how many you will get, but here's the method you will use: Just do your first set and stop about 1-2 reps before failure. Your goal is to have it so that your third set of diamond push-ups leaves you 1 rep short of failure. This is kind of tough to explain in writing so watch video #8 on www.CalisthenicsTribe.com.

Workout: BOOM/12/12/12/12 + Tricep Dips 8/8/BOOM(Wednesday)

This workout is where you are going to try to hit your 30 push-ups to pass on to level 4. You're going to BOOM it and try to hit your 30 push-ups on the first set, and then do 4 sets of 12 afterwards. After that, you just need to hit 3 sets of tricep dips, except they will be harder this time around. Instead of having your feet on the ground, they will be elevated on another chair (see picture below). This workout is essentially your weekly test to see if you can make it to level 4. If you can hit 30 push-ups on the first set, you're ready to go!

Tricep Dips (2 Chairs)
Start Position

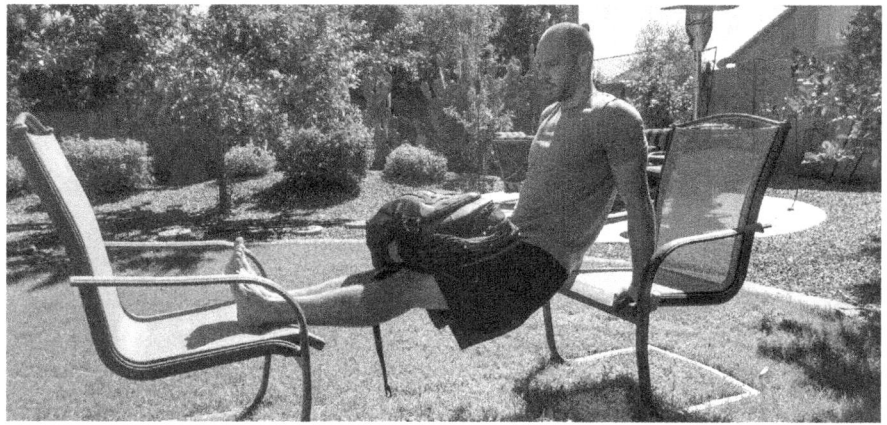

(Ignore the backpack for now, only use bodyweight)

End Position

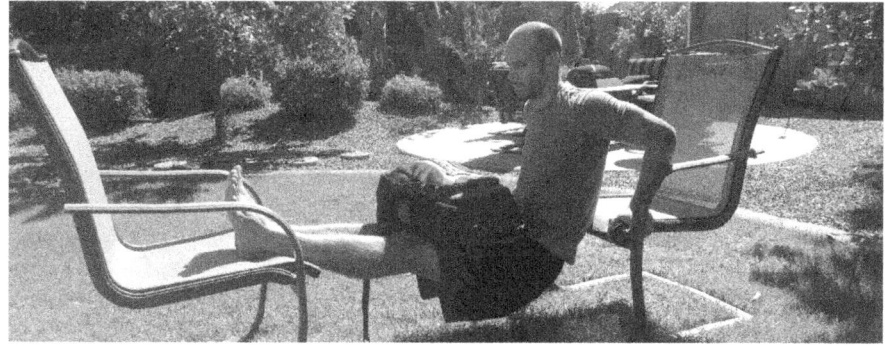

(Again, ignore backpack)

<u>Rest Periods</u>

Monday and Friday Workout
2 minutes for the Weighted Push-ups
2 minutes for the Diamond Push-ups

Wednesday Workout
1.5 minutes for the BOOM and 4x12 Push-ups
1.5 minutes for the Tricep Dips

Level 3 Completion Requirement: 30 full push-ups

Level 3 Sample Plan

Week 1

Day	Exercise 1		Exercise 2
1	Weighted Push-ups Set 1: 6 Set 2: 6 Set 3: 6		Diamond Push-ups Set 1: 8 Set 2: 8 Set 3: 8
2	Push-ups BOOM: 22 *New Record* Set 2: 12 Set 3: 12 Set 4: 12 Set 5: 12		Tricep Dips Set 1: 8 Set 2: 8 Set 3: 8
3	Weighted Push-ups Set 1: 6 Set 2: 6 Set 3: 7 *New Record*		Diamond Push-ups Set 1: 8 Set 2: 8 Set 3: 9 *New Record*

Week 2

Day	Exercise 1		Exercise 2
1	Weighted Push-ups Set 1: 6 Set 2: 6 Set 3: 9 *New Record*		Diamond Push-ups Set 1: 8 Set 2: 8 Set 3: 10 *New Record*
2	Push-ups BOOM: 24 *New Record* Set 2: 12 Set 3: 12 Set 4: 12 Set 5: 12		Tricep Dips Set 1: 8 Set 2: 8 Set 3: 10 *New Record*
3	**Added Weight** Weighted Push-ups Set 1: 6 Set 2: 6 Set 3: 6		Diamond Push-ups Set 1: 8 Set 2: 8 Set 3: 11 *New Record*

Week 3

Day	Exercise 1		Exercise 2
1	Weighted Push-ups Set 1: 6 Set 2: 6 Set 3: 7 *New Record*		Diamond Push-ups Set 1: 8 Set 2: 8 Set 3: 12 *New Record*
2	Push-ups BOOM: 27 *New Record* Set 2: 12 Set 3: 12 Set 4: 12 Set 5: 12		Tricep Dips Set 1: 8 Set 2: 8 Set 3: 11 *New Record*
3	Weighted Push-ups Set 1: 6 Set 2: 6 Set 3: 8 *New Record*		Added Weight Diamond Push-ups Set 1: 8 Set 2: 8 Set 3: 8

Week 4

Day	Exercise 1		Exercise 2
1	Added Weight Weighted Push-ups Set 1: 6 Set 2: 6 Set 3: 6		Diamond Push-ups Set 1: 8 Set 2: 8 Set 3: 9 *New Record*
2	Push-ups BOOM: 30 *New Record* Set 2: 12 Set 3: 12 Set 4: 12 Set 5: 12		Tricep Dips Set 1: 8 Set 2: 8 Set 3: 12 *New Record*
3	Weighted Push-ups Set 1: 6 Set 2: 6 Set 3: 8 *New Record*		Diamond Push-ups Set 1: 8 Set 2: 8 Set 3: 10 *New Record*

Chapter 4 - Level 4

Badge Head on over to the website and claim your level 3 badge!

Level 4 Workouts

Monday - Pseudo Planche Push-ups 3xBOOM + Weighted Diamond Push-ups 8/8/BOOM
Tuesday - Off
Wednesday - BOOM/15/15/15/15 + Weighted Tricep Dips 8/8/BOOM
Thursday - Off
Friday - 6/6/BOOM Weighted Push-ups 3xBOOM+ Weighted Diamond Push-ups 8/8/BOOM
Saturday - Off
Sunday - Off

Workout: Pseudo Planche Push-ups 3xBOOM+ Weighted Diamond Push-ups 8/8/BOOM (Monday and Friday)

Pseudo Planche Push-ups

Alright you're probably getting to the point where you don't have enough weight to stuff in your backpack to keep you in a low rep range, so now you are going to do something called a pseudo planche push-up.

They are quite a bit harder than regular push-ups, and you may not be able to do that many in the beginning weeks, but stick with it and you'll be doing more in no time. That progress will transfer over big time to regular push-ups.

Check out the coming pictures and video for the form.

Start Position

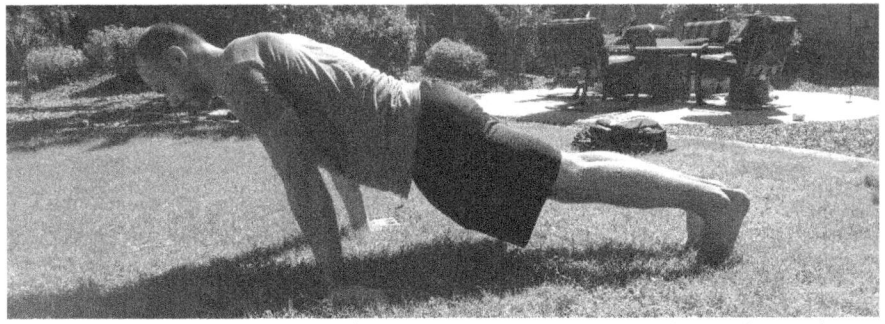

(Hands turned out so fingers are pointing to the side and slightly back. Hands positioned about shoulder width apart even with the stomach area)

End Position

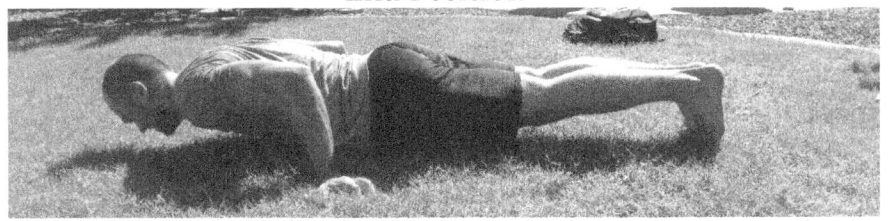

(Body should come forward and down, back stays straight)

Wrong End Position

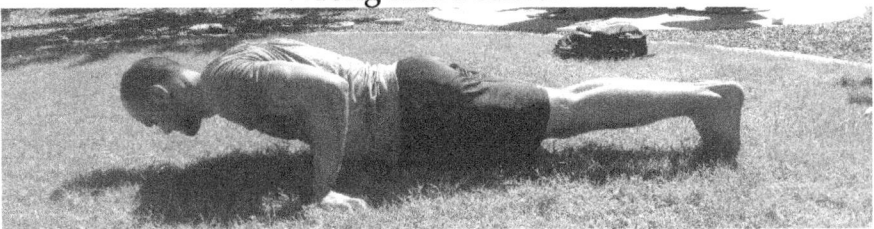

(In this position, you can see I only came straight down without leaning forward, which is incorrect.)

Similar to how you did the static holds you did in Level 1, you are going to just try to improve your total every time, so you will do a BOOM set as each of the 3 sets. Write down your total and try to beat it the next time you do pseudo planche push-ups. Watch video #9 if you would like a demonstration of the correct form.

Weighted Diamond Push-ups

For the diamond push-ups, we are doing the same thing as in level 3, except adding just a bit of weight (backpack). Rep scheme is 8/8/BOOM.

Workout: BOOM/15/15/15/15 + Weighted Tricep Dips 8/8/BOOM (Wednesday)

This workout is essentially the same as the one from level 3, except we've increased the reps after the BOOM to account for your improvement, and we are also going to add some weight to your tricep dips. Place something on your lap that makes it tough for you to get a single set of 10-12 reps, and then bust out 3 sets 8/8/BOOM style.

Weighted Tricep Dips

Start Position

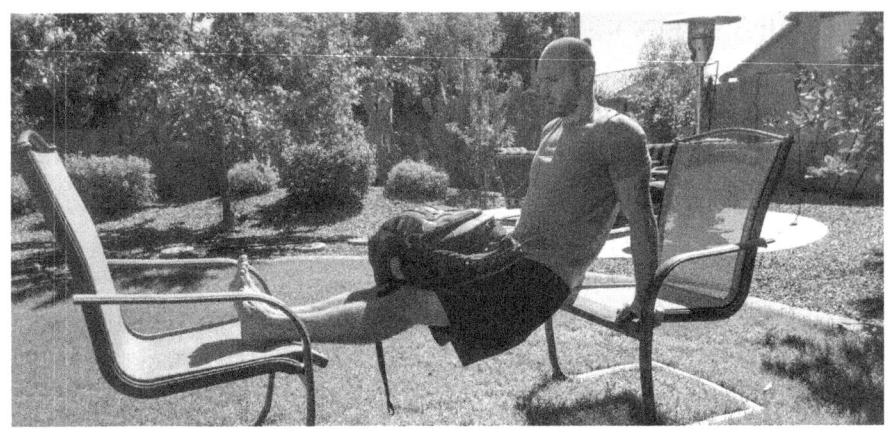

(Same picture from before, but now I want you to actually use the backpack for added weight)

End Position

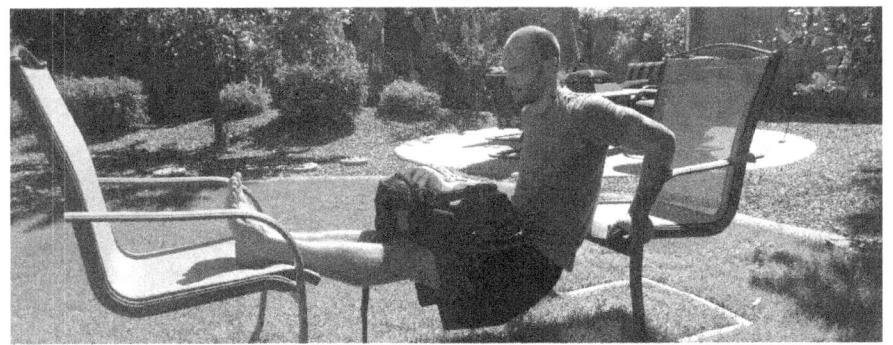

Rest Periods

Monday and Friday Workout
2.5 minutes for the Pseudo-Planche Push-ups
2 minutes for the Weighted Diamond Push-ups

Wednesday Workout
1.5 minutes for the BOOM and 4x15 Push-ups
1.5 minutes for the Weighted Tricep Dips

Level 4 Completion Requirement: 40 full push-ups

Level 4 Sample Plan

Week 1

Day	Exercise 1		Exercise 2
1	Pseudo-Planche Push-ups Set 1: 3 Set 2: 2 Set 3: 2 Total: 7		Weighted Diamond Push-ups Set 1: 8 Set 2: 8 Set 3: 8
2	Push-ups Set 1: 32 *New Record* Set 2: 15 Set 3: 15 Set 4: 15 Set 5: 15		Weighted Tricep Dips Set 1: 8 Set 2: 8 Set 3: 8
3	Pseudo-Planche Push-ups Set 1: 4 Set 2: 2 Set 3: 2 Total: 8 *New Record*		Weighted Diamond Push-ups Set 1: 8 Set 2: 8 Set 3: 9 *New Record*

Week 2

Day	Exercise 1		Exercise 2
1	Pseudo-Planche Push-ups Set 1: 4 Set 2: 3 Set 3: 2 Total: **9** *New Record*		Weighted Diamond Push-ups Set 1: 8 Set 2: 8 Set 3: 10 *New Record*
2	Push-ups Set 1: 35 *New Record* Set 2: 15 Set 3: 15 Set 4: 15 Set 5: 15		Weighted Tricep Dips Set 1: 8 Set 2: 8 Set 3: 9 *New Record*
3	Pseudo-Planche Push-ups Set 1: 5 Set 2: 3 Set 3: 3 Total: **11** *New Record*		Weighted Diamond Push-ups Set 1: 8 Set 2: 8 Set 3: 11 *New Record*

Week 3

Day	Exercise 1		Exercise 2
1	Pseudo-Planche Push-ups Set 1: 5 Set 2: 4 Set 3: 3 Total: **12** *New Record*		Added Weight Weighted Diamond Push-ups Set 1: 8 Set 2: 8 Set 3: 8
2	Push-ups Set 1: 37 *New Record* Set 2: 15 Set 3: 15 Set 4: 15 Set 5: 15		Weighted Tricep Dips Set 1: 8 Set 2: 8 Set 3: 10 *New Record*
3	Pseudo-Planche Push-ups Set 1: 6 Set 2: 5 Set 3: 4 Total: **15** *New Record*		Weighted Diamond Push-ups Set 1: 8 Set 2: 8 Set 3: 9 *New Record*

Week 4

Day	Exercise 1		Exercise 2
1	Pseudo-Planche Push-ups Set 1: 7 Set 2: 6 Set 3: 4 Total: 17 *New Record*		Weighted Diamond Push-ups Set 1: 8 Set 2: 8 Set 3: 10 *New Record*
2	Push-ups Set 1: 39 *New Record* Set 2: 15 Set 3: 15 Set 4: 15 Set 5: 15		Weighted Tricep Dips Set 1: 8 Set 2: 8 Set 3: 11 *New Record*
3	Push-ups Set 1: 40 **FULL PUSH-UPS** Set 2: 15 Set 3: 15 Set 4: 15 Set 5: 15 *Pass*		Weighted Diamond Push-ups Set 1: 8 Set 2: 8 Set 3: 11 *New Record*

Chapter 5 - Level 5

Badge Head on over to the website and receive your level 4 badge!

Level 5 Workouts

Monday - Weighted Planche Push-ups 5/5/BOOM + Weighted Decline Push-ups 8/8/BOOM
Tuesday - Off
Wednesday - BOOM/4x Power 12's + Weighted Tricep Dips 8/8/BOOM
Thursday - Off
Friday - Weighted Planche Push-ups 5/5/BOOM + Weighted Decline Push-ups 3x8
Saturday - Off
Sunday - Off

Workout: 6/6/BOOM Weighted Decline Push-ups 3x5 + Weighted Diamond Push-ups 1 Rep Short of Failure (Monday Only)

We're at the home stretch, and it's time to step our game up and give it that final push. The Monday and Friday workouts contain two very tough variations of the push-up, the weighted pseudo planche push-up and the weighted decline push-up.

Weighted Pseudo Planche Push-ups

You already know how to do the pseudo planche push-ups, but you will need to wear the weighted backpack this time around. Make sure you pack enough weight so that you can only get about 5 reps, and then BOOM out that 3rd set. Once you are able to get 8 reps on the last set with the current weight, reset to 5 reps with more weight.

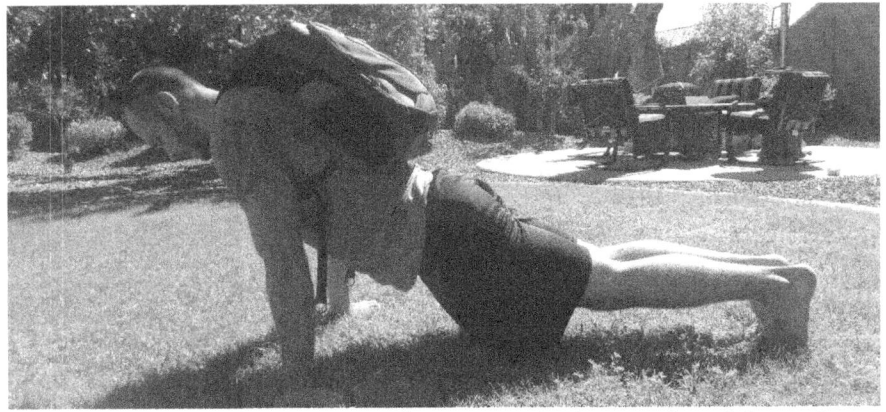

Start Position

(Hands turned out again, fingers pointing to the side and slightly backwards)

End Position

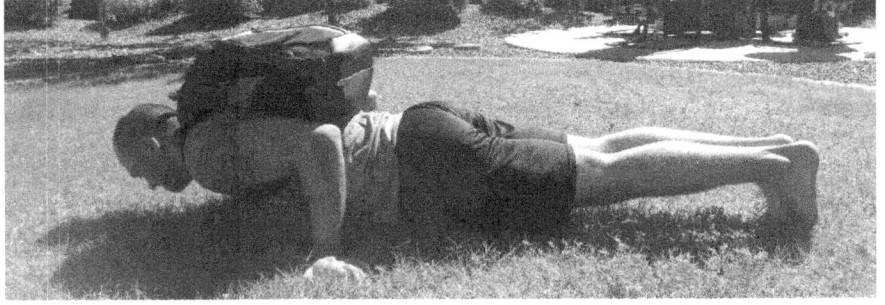

(Remember to lean forward as you come down)

<u>Weighted Decline Push-ups</u>

For the weighted decline push-ups, find something that will elevate your feet about 12 inches off the floor. If you'll remember that incline push-ups made push-ups easier, decline push-ups have the opposite effect, making them harder. You're just going to pick a weight that only allows you to do about 8 reps by the 3rd set, and then 8/8/BOOM it.

Start Position

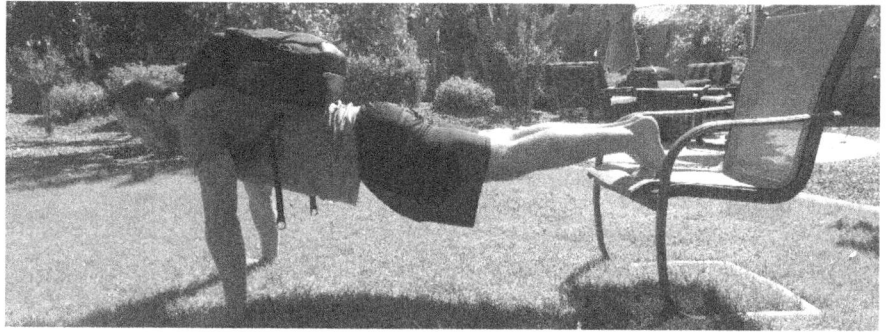

(Feet elevated on a chair or something about that high, hands just outside of shoulder width.)

End Position

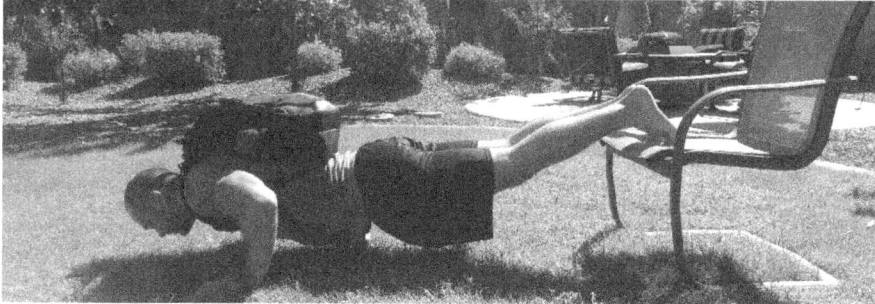

(Lower yourself just as you would for a regular push-up.)

Workout: BOOM/4x Power 12's + Weighted Tricep Dips (Wednesday)

Alright we've got some new stuff here. Your first set should be a BOOM to test you for the BIG 50. Write down whatever your BOOM turned out to be, and then move on to Power 12's.

Power 12's

Power 12's are push-ups with some added oomph, or plyometric push-ups. They are essentially clap push-ups, but you don't have to clap if you don't want to—just producing enough force to get your hands off the ground is enough. They are called Power 12's simply because you're going to do 12 of them. You will do 4 sets of Power 12's.

Start Position

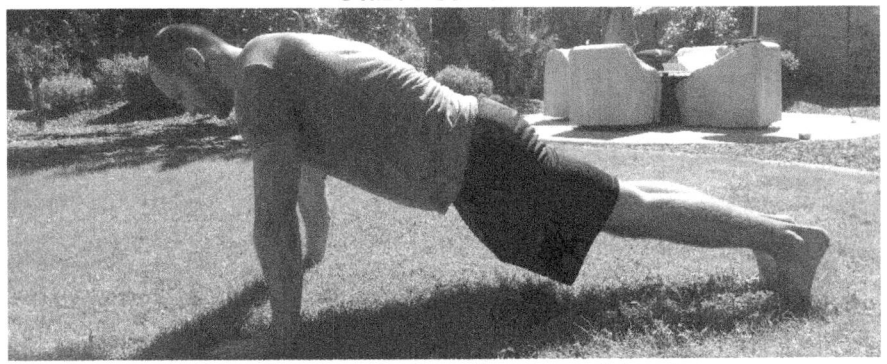

(Regular starting push-up position.)

Middle Position

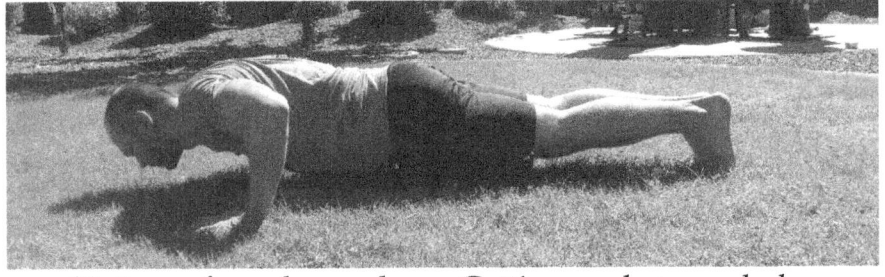

(Bottom of regular push-up. Getting ready to explode upwards.)

End Position

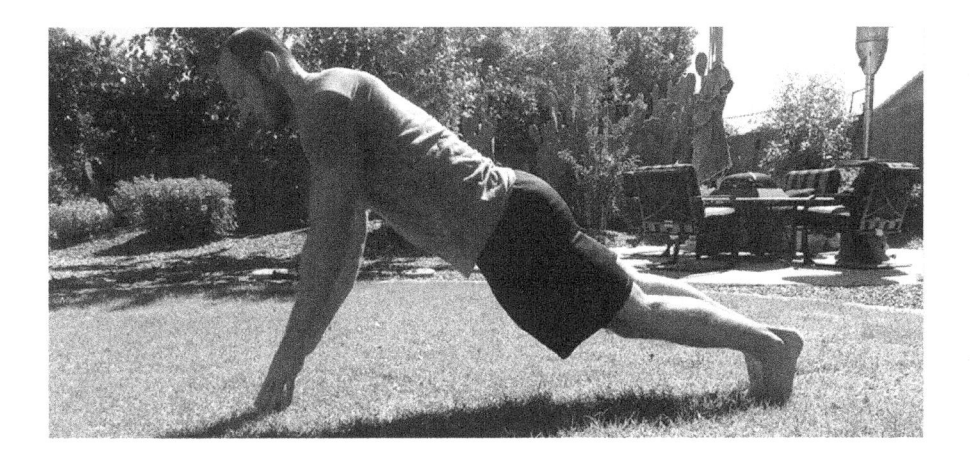

Weighted Tricep Dips

Then you'll move on to the weighted tricep dips again. Try to increase the weight a little bit from Level 4. Pick a weight that allows you to do 3 sets of 8 reps to start out.

Rest Periods

Monday and Friday Workout
2.5 minutes for the Weighted Pseudo-Planche Push-ups
2.5 minutes for the Weighted Decline Push-ups

Wednesday Workout
1.5 minutes for the BOOM and Power 12's
1.5 minutes for the Weighted Tricep Dips

Level 5 Completion Requirement: *50* full push-ups

Level 5 Sample Plan

Week 1

Day	Exercise 1		Exercise 2
1	Weighted Pseudo-Planche Push-ups Set 1: 5 Set 2: 5 Set 3: 5		Weighted Decline Push-ups Set 1: 8 Set 2: 8 Set 3: 8
2	Push-ups 43: *New Record* Set 1: Power 12's Set 2: Power 12's Set 3: Power 12's Set 4: Power 12's		Weighted Tricep Dips Set 1: 8 Set 2: 8 Set 3: 8
3	Weighted Pseudo-Planche Push-ups Set 1: 5 Set 2: 5 Set 3: 6 *New Record*		Weighted Decline Push-ups Set 1: 8 Set 2: 8 Set 3: 9 *New Record*

Week 2

Day	Exercise 1		Exercise 2
1	Weighted Pseudo-Planche Push-ups Set 1: 5 Set 2: 5 Set 3: 7 *New Record*		Weighted Decline Push-ups Set 1: 8 Set 2: 8 Set 3: 10 *New Record*
2	Push-ups: 45 *New Record* Set 1: Power 12's Set 2: Power 12's Set 3: Power 12's Set 4: Power 12's		Weighted Tricep Dips Set 1: 8 Set 2: 8 Set 3: 9 *New Record*
3	Weighted Pseudo-Planche Push-ups Set 1: 5 Set 2: 5 Set 3: 8 *New Record*		Weighted Decline Push-ups Set 1: 8 Set 2: 8 Set 3: 11 *New Record*

Week 3

Day	Exercise 1		Exercise 2
1	Added Weight Weighted Pseudo-Planche Push-ups Set 1: 5 Set 2: 5 Set 3: 5		Weighted Decline Push-ups Set 1: 8 Set 2: 8 Set 3: 12 *New Record*
2	Push-ups: 47 *New Record* Set 1: Power 12's Set 2: Power 12's Set 3: Power 12's Set 4: Power 12's		Weighted Tricep Dips Set 1: 8 Set 2: 8 Set 3: 10 *New Record*
3	Weighted Pseudo-Planche Push-ups Set 1: 5 Set 2: 5 Set 3: 6 *New Record*		Added Weight Weighted Decline Push-ups Set 1: 8 Set 2: 8 Set 3: 8

Week 4

Day	Exercise 1		Exercise 2
1	Weighted Pseudo-Planche Push-ups Set 1: 5 Set 2: 5 Set 3: 7 *New Record*		Weighted Decline Push-ups Set 1: 5 Set 2: 5 Set 3: 9 *New Record*
2	Push-ups: **50** Set 1: Power 12's Set 2: Power 12's Set 3: Power 12's Set 4: Power 12's *Pass*		Weighted Tricep Dips Set 1: 8 Set 2: 8 Set 3: 11 *New Record*
3	Weighted Pseudo-Planche Push-ups Set 1: 5 Set 2: 5 Set 3: 8 *New Record*		Weighted Decline Push-ups Set 1: 8 Set 2: 8 Set 3: 10 *New Record*

Now go on and collect your 50 Push-Up Challenge Badge!

Once you are able to BOOM out the BIG 50, you've done it!

That wasn't so hard now, was it? If you are looking to continue doing bodyweight exercises, Calisthenics Tribe is designed specifically for that. I will have posts about how to progress from each bodyweight or calisthenic exercise, along with other tips about diet, motivation, and anything fitness related.

Now, head on over to CalisthenicsTribe.com to claim your 50 Push-up Master badge!

Made in the USA
Monee, IL
03 March 2020